THE VALLEY

THE VALLEY

Joan MacLeod

Talonbooks

Talonbooks
278 East First Avenue, Vancouver, British Columbia, Canada v5T 1A6
www.talonbooks.com

First printing: 2014

Typeset in Adobe Caslon

Printed and bound in Canada on 100% post-consumer recycled paper
Cover illustration: KARO Group

Talonbooks gratefully acknowledges the financial support of the Canada Council for the Arts, the Government of Canada through the Canada Book Fund, and the Province of British Columbia through the British Columbia Arts Council and the Book Publishing Tax Credit.

Rights to produce *The Valley*, in whole or in part, in any medium by any group, amateur or professional, are retained by the author. Interested persons are requested to contact Pam Winter at the Gary Goddard Agency, 149 Church Street, 2nd Floor, Toronto, Ontario M5B 1Y4; tel.: (416) 928-0299; email: pam@garygoddardagency.com

Library and Archives Canada Cataloguing in Publication

MacLeod, Joan, 1954–, author
        The valley / Joan MacLeod.

A play.
Issued in print and electronic formats.
ISBN 978-0-88922-846-7 (pbk.).—ISBN 978-0-88922-847-4 (epub)

        I. Title.

PS8575.L4645V34 2014   C812'.54   C2014-900469-9
                                                                      C2014-900470-2

The Valley premiered on March 6, 2013, at Alberta Theatre Projects, Calgary, as part of the Enbridge playRites Festival of New Canadian Plays, with the following cast and crew:

Connor	Zachary Dugan
Dan	Kyle Jespersen
Janie	Erin MacKinnon
Sharon	Esther Purves-Smith

Director	Linda Moore
Set, lighting, and projection designer	Scott Reid
Costume designer	April Viczko
Composer and sound designer	Jonathan Lewis
Fight director	Laryssa Yanchak
Stage manager	Johanne Deleeuw
Dramaturg	Laurel Green
Assistant set, lighting, and projection designer	Erin Gruber
Assistant stage manager	Oliver Armstrong
Assistant stage manager	Patti Neice
Assistant costume designer	Juli Elkiw

A revised version of *The Valley* opened on November 13, 2013, at Tarragon Theatre, Toronto, with the following cast and crew:

Connor	Colin Mercer
Dan	Ian Lake
Janie	Michelle Monteith
Sharon	Susan Coyne

Director	Richard Rose
Set and lighting designer	Graeme S. Thomson
Costume designer	Charlotte Dean
Composer and sound designer	Todd Charlton
Fight director	John Stead
Stage manager	Marie Fewer
Assistant director	Maria Milisavljevic
Apprentice stage manager	Robin Munro
Assistant set and lighting designer	Nick Andison

Acknowledgements

The first act of *The Valley* was written at the Stratford Festival's 2010 Playwrights Retreat. Thank you, Bob White, for the invitation and support. The first complete draft was written and developed at the Banff Centre as part of the 2012 Playwrights Colony. This colony has been instrumental to the development of all my stage plays and once again I thank the centre profusely.

Thank you, Linda Moore, and the dedicated cast and crew at Alberta Theatre Projects, for contributing so much to the creation of this script; I am also indebted to Richard Rose and the cast and crew at Tarragon.

Thank you to my early readers – Daniel MacIvor, Don Hannah, Bill Gaston, Sally Stubbs, and psychiatric nurse Ingrid Currey.

Thank you to Constable Roger Reinson of the Calgary Police Service and to the Vancouver Police Department for its documentary series *The Beat*.

Thank you, Lorna Jackson, for lending me Andrew Solomon's *The Noonday Demon: An Atlas of Depression* – a phenomenal read that was instrumental in this play's creation.

Thank you, Bill and Ana, once more, for letting me fly away from you too many times to work on this play.

Finally, thank you, Vicki Stroich, Vanessa Porteous, Dianne Goodman, and all the good folk at Alberta Theatre Projects who worked at the playRites Festival during the past twenty-eight years. It was a joy to be part of it every time.

Characters

Connor: eighteen years old
Dan: thirty years old, police officer
Janie: twenty-five years old, Dan's wife
Sharon: fifty years old, Connor's mother

Settings

Sharon and Connor's house
Dan and Janie's house
The police station
SkyTrain stations

Performance Note

In monologue and when directly addressing the audience, characters sometimes stand ninety degrees apart at points around the edge of an invisible circle. From here, characters also sometimes address one another, exchange a look, or share an action when bridging the end of one scene to the beginning of the next. These moments of connection are important.

Scenes in the first act take place in the past and build toward the SkyTrain incident. In the second act, they occur after the incident and build toward the healing circle at the end of the play. The healing circle exists in another reality or on another plane that is not rooted in the realism of the other scenes.

The play unfolds over eight months, from late August one year to late April the next. There should be a sense of fluid transition between scenes, back and forth between past to present, and from one location to another.

Act One

Lights up on CONNOR.

CONNOR

Encounters with the police, number one. I went to this party. There were hundreds of people there because the guy's parents were away for the weekend. He'd moved most of the furniture out of the house and into the garage because he didn't want anything to get wrecked. He was trying to be responsible. But when the cops showed up they didn't even care. They still made everyone go home.

Number two. Sierra. We went to grad with each other because you had to go with whoever they said, so no one would feel left out. I didn't know Sierra. At all. She was tall. She talked – a lot. She was wearing this silver dress that she bought at Winners. *Why pay full price when you can go to Winners?* I don't know. I'd never been to Winners but for some reason everything Sierra said made fantastic sense to me.

So we go on this cruise in English Bay and eat pot cookies that Sierra and her friend Nina have made. Sierra, she never stops talking – while we eat at the buffet, while we watch the stars come out … She's going to move to the Island because Vancouver sucks. She's going to study early childhood education. Or massage therapy. Or she'll open a bakery – for dogs.

I am supposed to phone my dad for a ride when we get back in but I don't. Sierra and me go to the beach with Nina and her guy.

We do some E and wait for the sun to come up. I put my jacket on the sand so Sierra's dress doesn't get wrecked. Her toes are painted silver and are sticking out through the end of her pantyhose. I had sex before, when I was in grade ten. But this is different.

The edge of the beach … it's the edge of the world, the edge of the whole universe. There are birds making noise. Sierra, she's making noise too. A lot of noise.

And then all of a sudden this guy comes loping down the beach. Sierra tells me to get off her. Now. The guy's a cop. He watches – like really watches – while we pull on our clothes.

Then he wants to see our IDs. *You don't need ID to sit on a fucking beach!* That's what we say to each other. Later. The cop dumps out Sierra's purse. The drugs are all gone. Consumed.

He asks us if this is our grad and when we tell him yes he wishes us good luck in our future. Then he heads off for the next group down the beach.

Except everything was wrecked. We weren't high anymore. The girls wanted to go home. Sierra's face was puffy. Her Winners dress looked like shit.

I never liked cops. Even in grade six when they came to our school and dared us all to stay away from drugs. We just thought they were idiots.

Encounter number three. Last November. The Joyce Street SkyTrain station.

> *Pause.*

I don't know. You tell me. I don't remember.

> *Shift.*

Four months earlier. Two large suitcases wait by the door.
SHARON slips a letter into one of them. CONNOR
enters and SHARON tries hard to remain composed.

SHARON

Here we are! The big day!

CONNOR

If you get all weird and sad I'm going to call a taxi to take me to the airport right now.

SHARON

I said I'd drive you. I want to drive you.

CONNOR

I'll be home at Thanksgiving, Mum. It's only six weeks away.

SHARON

Did you pack your ski jacket? I looked up the weather forecast, for the year, in the *Farmer's Almanac*. It's supposed to be a mild winter there, but that's nothing like a mild winter here.

CONNOR

If I don't have a warm enough jacket I can go buy one. I'm not going to the Arctic. It's Calgary.

SHARON

You're positive about Calgary? With your marks I'll bet it's not too late to –

CONNOR

We're not getting into this again.

SHARON

I loved the University of Toronto. Every single minute of it. The classes, living in residence, the city.

CONNOR

I know, Mum. I want to go to Calgary.

SHARON

If you went to U of T, I could finally finish my master's. We could get a place, a two-bedroom in a house in the Annex.

CONNOR

NOT going to happen.

SHARON

Just think about it for next year … I'd cook good meals, help you with your essays, and if you had friends over I'd … I'd give you lots of space!

CONNOR

I wouldn't have any friends if I were living with my mother. I don't have any friends now and I live with you.

SHARON

That's not true! (*beat*) I read about this boy who lived in residence at UBC – he ate no vegetables, no fresh food for three months.

CONNOR

And I don't want to go to UBC. It'd be too much like high school all over again.

SHARON

That boy got scurvy.

CONNOR

So you want to come to university and live with me so that I don't get scurvy?

SHARON

And mono. Everyone ends up with mono in first year. The kissing disease!

CONNOR

Oh god –

SHARON

Sweetie, I just want to say –

CONNOR

I'm phoning Dad. I'll make him drive me to the airport.

SHARON

Going to university, one of the best parts is getting away from everyone you know. I get that.

CONNOR

Of course you do.

SHARON

I felt the very same way. Exactly.

CONNOR

Because you can identify with everything that's ever happened to me.

SHARON

That's right. It's a gift.

Do you have your old glasses in case the new ones break?

Shift.

Lights up on DAN.

DAN

First brush with the law? Kindergarten. Officer Something sitting with us in a circle on those little chairs. He was there to tell us about traffic safety, but us boys, we were all about the gun.

We wanted to see this officer's piece. We wanted to know how many people he killed per day. The teacher, she's trying to get things back on track. She doesn't want to make his visit all about the gun.

We'd made driver's licences that morning. Then we all got our turn behind the wheel of this pedal car that we tried to kill each other over on a daily basis. The officer pretended to pull us over.

5

So it was my turn. He asked me to haul out my licence … but this guy, I tell you, he had me in some sort of trance: the badge, the stick, even the buttons on his uniform – they made this impression on me. I couldn't move. The teacher tried to help me out. *Danny. What do you do when the policeman pulls you over?* And then I remembered what my dad did. My uncles too. *You hide your beer!*

High school. Run-in numero two. We got pulled over coming home from a lacrosse game. Eleven of us in this beat-up Buick. The driver's loaded. He got a suspension and the rest of us got to walk four miles home. Talk about getting off easy.

Janie read online that the Mother was going to release a victim impact statement to the press. Of course it isn't a real victim impact statement. It's just this thing she made up. A real victim impact statement is what real victims read in court before sentencing. Janie wanted me to call Riley – this guy I grew up with who's an editor with the *Sun* now – cut them off at the pass. I don't call Riley. There're protocols to follow. A guy doesn't just phone up the newspaper and start talking.

He looks toward SHARON.

The Mother here thinks the press is a courtroom. Her statement thing is all about how her son has always been the perfect kid. And how they've always been the perfect parents since the dawn of time. But I don't give a shit what she says. I really don't.

Shift.

Lights up on JANIE, three months earlier. She has just put baby Zeke to sleep. DAN enters.

JANIE

He didn't nap at all this morning. Then he finally passed out around five.

I spent hours trying to make the sides go higher on the crib. But I couldn't follow the directions. I even read them in French and then in what I think was Spanish. Then I was reading directions in some language with a weird alphabet but thinking maybe it's our alphabet and I'm so tired that I've forgotten what our alphabet looks like.

DAN

Zeke always sleeps like a baby for me. There's nothing to it. Down and out.

JANIE

Even in your line of work the chances of you being killed at home are still much greater than –

DAN kisses JANIE.

JANIE

Then I finally fell asleep. Or I think I fell asleep. I can't tell anymore if I'm asleep or awake. Maybe I'm asleep right now.

DAN

That'd be nice.

JANIE

What does that mean?

DAN

It means it would be nice for you and everybody involved if you could get more sleep. Why are you messing around with the crib?

JANIE

When I woke up this morning he was trying to sit up in it.

DAN

Zeke can sit up?

JANIE

He's trying to.

DAN

That's awesome. He is so awesome.

JANIE

He already wants to escape – run away from his stupid mother.

DAN

You just lower where the mattress is and then the sides are higher. Right?

Pause.

JANIE

Dan –

DAN

Janie.

JANIE

Don't push me. Don't push my buttons.

DAN

You don't have any buttons. You're hanging out in your pyjamas all day.

JANIE

They're yoga pants.

DAN

Those are not yoga pants. I'll fix the crib in the morning …
It took years and years to get my brother out of his crib.
Bozo was –

JANIE

Bobby.

DAN

– he was parked there in his crib beside the bunk beds, taking up half our room until he was, like, four. And he wouldn't give up his stroller until he broke the thing in half because he was so unbelievably big.

He looked like a gigantic hairless cat. And he cried constantly – a complete tyrant right from the start. Even then he was a nightmare. That just says it all, doesn't it?

JANIE

He was probably just colicky. I bet Zeke inherited that from your side of the family, from his uncle Bobby.

DAN

Twenty-nine years old and he's still colicky.

DAN starts to exit.

JANIE

That's nice. I'm desperate for someone to talk to all day and then you come home and don't want to talk to me.

DAN stops.

DAN

So talk. (*beat*) I hate leaving you guys every morning. I hate that he's asleep right now. I want to hang out with him.

JANIE

If you wake up Zeke I'll kill you.

DAN sits beside JANIE. She leans into him.

DAN

You've got to stop making threats against my person.

JANIE

I love your person.

When Jason and me were squatting in that A-frame, he'd go off to make a deal or lease a brand new Jeep Cherokee or beat the shit out of somebody. And I'd sit there on this mattress on the floor all day. Snow falling through the trees …

That's what being at home with Zeke is like … some of the time. It's … it's lonely.

DAN stands up.

JANIE

What? So that makes me an awful mother? Where are you going?

DAN

Outside. I'm going to work on the bike.

You know, when I get up I look at you and I look at Zeke and I know that I'm the luckiest guy in the world. When you get up you start making a list of everything that's wrong. And that stuff with Jason … Jesus, Janie. It's ancient history.

JANIE

I know that.

DAN

Good.

JANIE

Go. Go outside and play with your bike.

DAN

You sure?

JANIE

Go.

Shift.

Lights up on SHARON.

SHARON

Prior encounters with the police, number one. Woolco. My friend Susie and I got caught switching price tags. We wanted these belts that were $2.99 so we switched price tags with some bandanas that were $1.49. We didn't even really think of it as stealing.

Woolco wanted to set some sort of example so they called the police. The store detective marched the two of us, by the arm, right through the store and to this waiting police car for everyone to see. It was all very dramatic.

The two police officers didn't speak to us. They just drove us home. By some act of God my parents were out. So they just dropped us off. Case closed.

Later my parents found out from the neighbours that I'd arrived home under police escort. I told them I'd found a purse and turned it in, so the police had given me a ride home as a reward for being such an outstanding citizen. My god – the ability kids have to lie on the spot. It's spectacular.

Connor didn't have anything to do with the police – before. He was home with us all the time, holed up in his room. Even when he was fifteen years old he would've rather been writing.

Lights up on fifteen-year-old CONNOR at his laptop. He reads from his novel manuscript.

CONNOR

TO EXIST ON THE PLANET ZURCON, ONE REQUIRED THREE THINGS: OXYGEN, WATER, AND A PURE HEART. VASALON KNEW THAT HIS HEART WAS PURE. HE COULD FEEL IT BEATING AT ONE HUNDRED BEATS PER SECOND INSIDE HIS LARGE, STRONG CHEST.

THE PLANET WAS BROKEN INTO QUADRANTS AND FROM SPACE LOOKED LIKE A GIGANTIC SPINNING BEACH BALL. VASALON LIVED IN THE GREEN QUADRANT BECAUSE HIS BLOOD WAS GREEN – A NOBLE AND AWESOME COLOUR.

SHARON

Connor didn't have the opportunity to get into trouble.
He didn't live for the weekend the way I did at that age.

CONNOR

VASALON HAD BEEN ON HIS OWN FOR AS LONG AS
HE COULD REMEMBER. HE WAS BUT A YOUNG LAD
WHEN A FRAGMENT FROM A METEOR PIERCED HIS
MOTHER'S SKULL AND MADE HER BRAIN EXPLODE.

Lights out on CONNOR.

SHARON

Encounter number two. December 1995, when our Dodge
Caravan was stolen. You couldn't kill that van with a stick.
They found it submerged in the Fraser but it still ran another
four years.

Encounter number three. April 2004. My cellphone and I sit on
the curb beside a homeless person, who may or may not be
dead, and wait for the police to arrive. I realize this … this
gentleman is still alive when he pisses his pants, when he grabs
on to my arm and holds on and holds on. He holds on to me
during what really are the last moments of his life. That awful
smell, the curb, the garbage in the gutter.

Calling what finally showed up a policeman is completely
inaccurate. He was a police boy. He was a police boy with soft,
blond curls and blue, blue eyes. He kept apologizing to me
because this man had died right beside me. The police boy's
eyes were so bright that I was afraid he was going to burst out
crying …

Constable Mulano's eyes looked cold – the eyes of a reptile.
(*looks toward DAN*) *The Mother.* That's what he calls me. He
calls me the Mother because then he doesn't have to think of
me as a real human being.

Shift.

Two months earlier. Lights up on CONNOR, still half-asleep, staring at a place setting on the table. SHARON enters.

SHARON

It's … terrific that you're getting caught up on your sleep! I remember how exhausting first year can be. Especially these first couple of months.

CONNOR looks at his mother blankly.

SHARON

I can make you a turkey sandwich. Or if you still want breakfast there's bacon and eggs. There's cereal. Not just my cereal. There's Cheerios and Harvest Crunch. Sweetie?

CONNOR remains unresponsive.

SHARON

You must still be jet-lagged. Or it's the turkey drug making you sleepy. Even with the turkey drug I woke up again at three this morning. Except, for once, it wasn't just me rattling around in this house in the middle of the night … Are you finding school exhausting?

CONNOR

I find YOU exhausting.

SHARON

I'll get out the eggs.

CONNOR

I'm not hungry either.

SHARON

But you barely ate dinner last night. And you love Thanksgiving dinner.

CONNOR

It's, like, an hour away.

SHARON

What?

CONNOR

Calgary. It's an eighty-minute flight from Vancouver.
A one-hour time difference. I'm not jet-lagged. (*beat*) I dropped environmental studies.

SHARON

Why?

CONNOR

And philosophy. I wasn't … engaged.

SHARON

What does that mean?

CONNOR

It means it was all bullshit.

SHARON

Some of us didn't expect university to be entertaining. What are you taking instead of philosophy and environmental studies?

CONNOR

Writing. And astronomy.

SHARON

And English. I know that. What are you taking instead of philosophy and environmental studies?

CONNOR

Nothing.

SHARON

You're only taking three courses?

CONNOR

Did I say I was taking three courses?

SHARON

Connor –

CONNOR

I dropped environmental studies. And philosophy.

SHARON

You just said that.

CONNOR

And probably English. I'm thinking about dropping English.

SHARON

The novel study? Why would you do that? You couldn't wait to take that course –

CONNOR

Tess pranced down the rosy country lane with her fluttering bosom fluttering!

SHARON

Don't you dare make fun of Thomas Hardy! You know how much he means to me. (*beat*) If you go down below three courses you'll lose your scholarship money.

CONNOR

The books are so boring and … I can't finish any of them. I can hardly start them.

SHARON

Your dad won't be able to keep you on his medical if you drop below three courses. And if you think I'll ever get benefits at my job, you're sadly mistaken.

CONNOR

It's not my fault that you work in a bookstore. You don't have to work there.

SHARON

The point is why this is happening in the first place. Why are you dropping courses?

CONNOR

I haven't dropped English yet. I just haven't been for a while.

SHARON

Connor. Talk to me. What's going on?

CONNOR

Nothing.

SHARON

Your dad said you were having some issues with your roommate.

CONNOR

I don't have issues. Ethan has issues.

SHARON

How is creative writing going? Did you show your professor your books?

CONNOR

He doesn't have time to read novels. He has 135 students. He doesn't even have time to mark our assignments. The TA marks them.

SHARON

Would it help if I dropped him a note or I could –

CONNOR

You think I'm still in kindergarten.

SHARON

I'm just trying to figure out what happened to the young man who walked out the door six weeks ago and couldn't wait to start university. I'm really, really concerned about you.

CONNOR

Adverbs are weak words. Did you know that? You use adverbs all the time. *Completely. Utterly. Abominably.*

SHARON

Stop it.

CONNOR

Verily verily. Jesus Christ was King of the Adverbs. I'm going to tell that to Ethan the Mormon.

SHARON

Does your dad know you've dropped two courses? Connor. I'm talking to you –

CONNOR

I'm not going back.

SHARON

Excuse me?

CONNOR

You can't make me go back. I'll still get 50 percent on my tuition. I'll pay back everything I owe you. I mean it. Everything.

> *Pause.*

I'm sorry, Mum.

SHARON

What happened?

CONNOR

Nothing happened!

SHARON

A normal person doesn't suddenly decide after looking forward to something for years and years to give up all of a sudden and –

CONNOR

I should've taken a year off. A lot of people I know are taking a year off. Paul's in Fort McMurray making, like, twenty bucks an hour. I could do that. I should've done something like that. Just for this year.

SHARON

Paul didn't finish high school. He doesn't have the options, the opportunities you have in front of you.

CONNOR

Or that government thing where you go do volunteer work. I could help Inuits. Or salmon. I could help … something.

SHARON

If you were interested in volunteering, if that was your goal, then you should have been applying to different agencies and you should've been doing so, undoubtedly, in the spring.

CONNOR

Undoubtedly. Impossibly. Irretrievably. Dementedly.

SHARON

This is ridiculous!

CONNOR

Finally.

> *SHARON begins to exit.*

CONNOR

Ethan takes stuff from me. Pens. Pages from my notebook. He knows the password for my computer.

SHARON

There must be someone at the residence who you can talk to about that.

CONNOR

I'm not going back.

SHARON

I'll fly back with you and help sort this out.

CONNOR

Every single night, as soon as I've gone to bed, Ethan phones his girlfriend and talks to her for hours and hours and hours.

SHARON

We'll try again to get you a single room.

CONNOR

Would you fucking listen to me for once? I'm not going back!

Shift.

Lights up on JANIE.

JANIE

My mum was always calling the cops. PRE-Jason even. She believed in community policing way before it was ever invented.

Maybe there was a car parked outside our house that seemed suspicious because she'd never seen it before or the plates were from somewhere else or the driver was wearing a red hat. Maybe she wanted an expert opinion on whether or not my sister and I had been smoking dope. Maybe she was out of her mind – okay, understandably out of her mind – when her youngest daughter moved in with, you know, an asshole.

But the very first encounter with the police ... I'd have been maybe eight years old. Which would make Christine, my sister, thirteen. We broke a window in the basement. We were pushing our heads against the windowpane to see whether or not it would break. Our dad had taken off, vacated for good, maybe a month before. My mum freaked out about the window and she called the police. I thought she called them because she wanted to put us in jail, our own mother, and Christine probably promoted that version of things. But it was because it was after supper and everything was closed and Mum didn't know how to fix anything.

So this OPP came to our house. He was French. He had the accent going. Christine paraded around in her bikini while he boarded up the window.

Small-town stuff. A cop coming to fix an abandoned woman's
window …

Dan would do that. He would tell you that a good portion of
the calls he goes out on are about loneliness, about being alone.

All that stuff she's been saying about him? Wrong and wrong
again. Dan is this very loyal and … romantic individual. He has
this romantic soul. I don't. Maybe I did once but that's another
story. (*looks toward SHARON*) It's bullshit – what she's been
saying about Danny.

> *Shift.*

> *One month earlier. DAN is at home. JANIE enters.*

DAN

He just passed out. But not before putting up a good fight.
It's got to be exhausting carrying around such a big bean all day.
Do you think Zeke's got an especially enormous head?

JANIE

Babies have big heads. He's normal.

DAN

He's para-supernormal. He's amazing. Wanna make
another one?

JANIE

You mean right now?

DAN

If you say so.

JANIE

I'm kind of wiped.

DAN

Let's plan to start trying again for number two. It's easier to have them closer together.

JANIE

Easier for who?

DAN

That's what everyone says.

Beat.

JANIE

Actually I was thinking about going back to work. Maybe just half days – maybe just a couple of days a week.

DAN

When he's two.

JANIE

I was thinking more like now. I can get a pump.

DAN

What?

JANIE

And that Vietnamese lady in the first building, by the playground – she takes in kids. And she has experience with babies. Lots of babies. It's not a licensed daycare but it's good. All the mothers here say it's good. Her patio backs right onto the playground.

DAN

He's not going to the Vietnamese lady. Jesus, Janie. A goddamn pump?

JANIE

We could use the money.

DAN

He's not even six months old. Dennis stayed home until Emma was three. What's wrong with you?

JANIE

A lot. You knew that when you signed on. You said none of it mattered.

DAN

I didn't know you wouldn't want to stay home with your own baby.

DAN exits.

Lights up on CONNOR. JANIE looks toward him.

Shift.

CONNOR sits at his laptop, finishing off a joint.

CONNOR

VASALON IS TURNING TO ICE. HE NOTICES IT FIRST IN HIS FEET — HIS TOES BECOMING CLEAR AND BRITTLE, HIS HANDS CLOSE TO SHATTERING. EVERYTHING IS COLD.

HE KNOWS THAT IF HE MOVES EVEN AN INCH, CRACKS WILL FORM UP HIS LEGS AND SPINE. HIS HEART IS FROZEN, HIS SOUL AN ENDLESS RAVINE COVERED IN SNOW.

CONNOR is interrupted by rapping on the door. Lights up on SHARON, out on JANIE.

CONNOR

Fuck.

CONNOR closes his laptop.

SHARON

(*through the door*) I appreciate that you're looking for work online BUT there might be something tacked up in a window or in one of the weeklies that isn't on the computer BUT it just may be the perfect job. You won't know about it though if you just keep holed up in your room.

Beat.

It's been nearly a month now.

Beat.

There's a BIG WIDE RAINY WORLD out there!

Beat.

Connor? Could you please at least acknowledge that you are in your room? That you are listening? That I am not talking to a brick wall?

CONNOR

You are not talking to a brick wall.

SHARON

And perhaps your expectations given your lack of experience are a tiny bit high.

CONNOR flicks the joint away.

SHARON

Smoking grass every day isn't going to help either. Look. I know you are capable of doing anything you put your mind to. Anything. Both your dad and I feel that way. But maybe it would be a good idea to have a shower, put on some clean clothes, and talk to a counsellor – an employment counsellor. Maybe it would be a good idea to talk to a regular counsellor too – about Calgary, about your having to come home.

Pause.

Did you know that one in four university students experiences prolonged periods of anxiety or depression? Especially young males. Especially in first year when it's their first time away from home. It isn't anything to be ashamed of.

There was a well-worn path between my residence and the counselling centre when I was at U of T. I took full advantage of –

CONNOR throws open the door.

CONNOR

If you tell me that you know how I feel, how THIS feels …

If you even insinuate for one second that you have a fucking clue what it's like to be me, here, now, living this shitty stupid life. IF you try and do that one more time – I'm going to kill myself!

SHARON

DON'T say that!

CONNOR

I mean it.

SHARON

You say many, many things to me. And sometimes they are hurtful, hateful things but I know that deep down it's … it's … AWESOME that we can have open communication. But … YOU CANNOT SAY THAT TO ME!

CONNOR

Okay.

SHARON

Okay.

Pause.

CONNOR

In Calgary, when I got up to pee in the middle of the night – when I walked on the carpet down the hall – sparks came out from under my heels. I'm not kidding.

SHARON

That happened when we were in Jasper too – it's the dryness.

CONNOR

Then I'd go up on the roof of the residence and even when it was pitch-black … the air … the air was full of static. Charged up. And the Rockies – they would reveal themselves to me.

SHARON

What are you doing on the roof of the residence at night? (*beat*) Connor?

CONNOR

I got a job.

SHARON

You did?

CONNOR

Yeah. I did. I got a job.

SHARON

That's terrific. That is wonderful news. Why didn't you tell me?

CONNOR

It's with Student Painters.

SHARON

Student Painters! I can see you with Student Painters. I can see you clearly.

CONNOR

I have eliminated adverbs from my speech.

> *Beat.*

SHARON

When do you start your job?

CONNOR

Next Tuesday.

SHARON

So it wasn't an issue for anyone there that you aren't a student right now? At this particular point in time?

CONNOR

I didn't have an interview with some executive in his office. They didn't even ask for references. I filled out this thing online. Besides you don't need to be a student to deliver flyers.

SHARON

You're delivering flyers for Student Painters! You mean door to door?

CONNOR

No, Mother. I'm going to hire a plane and drop them from the sky. Yes, door to door. That's what delivering flyers is. In what universe would delivering flyers mean anything other than going door to door?

Shift.

DAN is getting dressed for work. This is the first time we see him onstage in uniform.

DAN

Zeke has these long, flat, amazing feet. They're all padded underneath. We all start out in this world flat-footed, which I didn't know. Janie told me that, because she's always skipping ahead in the baby book – *What to Expect at Twenty-Four Months.* That's when the arch becomes something you can see.

I can spend way too much time thinking about what's happening inside my son's feet. How right now the bones are growing, doing their thing. I thought a baby would be boring because other babies are boring. I tell Janie it's cheating to skip ahead in the baby book. Zeke at five months is the place to be.

Zeke from *Ezekiel.* It means "God will strengthen you."

Lights up on SHARON, ninety degrees away
from DAN.

SHARON

Connor. Lover of Wolves.

DAN

Ezekiel was an Old Testament guy. I don't know much about him.

SHARON looks toward DAN.

SHARON

What to expect at eighteen years and three months. Your child will split in two. His first psychotic break.

Tuesday. Late afternoon. On the very first day of his very first job. Joyce SkyTrain station.

DAN bangs his locker closed. He's ready for work.

DAN

I hate Joyce Station. It's got a place of honour on the shit list. It's a shit way to start a twelve-hour shift.

Lights up on JANIE, ninety degrees from SHARON.

DAN

Someone in the third car had pushed the alarm. Texts were coming into the emergency dispatcher from the people in the car: FLIPPD OUT * MAN W WEAPON * ATTACKD. We're waiting for the train to pull into the station.

SHARON

They'd already called for backup. They were having some difficulty keeping everyone away from the track.

JANIE

You'd think that when people see two cops, hands on weapons, telling everyone to keep clear, that something might be going on that's more important than getting home for dinner.

Something more important than cracking a beer and watching the hockey game.

SHARON

Even before the train pulled in, things were getting out of hand.

DAN

We couldn't keep the platform clear because it's rush hour. Because people are stupid. Then this old lady with a shopping cart starts yammering away at Dennis in Chinese and we got separated – me and Dennis. That wasn't anyone's fault. She's a good partner. And then the train comes –

> *Lights up on CONNOR, who completes the circle. He holds a sword-like object and is slicing the air all around him.*
>
> *SFX: The train arriving.*
>
> *SFX: An announcement. "This is Joyce-Collingwood Station. The next train to arrive on the inbound platform is for Waterfront Station."*

DAN

The doors open and there's this kid.

SHARON

Connor …

DAN

He's a fucking mess. Everyone is trying to stand as far away from him as possible. There's a direct path between the kid and me; he's right there in the middle of the car. The alarms are going off in the station but it feels quiet. Because nobody is talking. The kid's got something in his hand.

JANIE

A weapon.

SHARON

A so-called weapon –

DAN

He is brandishing the weapon. By that I mean he's swinging it round and round, keeping the passengers at bay.

Lights brighten. CONNOR and DAN look at each other for the first time. Everyone takes a step toward the centre of the circle.

DAN

Police …

The circle dissolves. We go back to that day in the SkyTrain station, CONNOR swinging what looks like a homemade sword, DAN taking a couple of steps toward him. Now DAN is all business.

DAN

Weapon on the floor.

CONNOR

It's a light baton.

DAN

ON THE FLOOR! NOW!

CONNOR stops swinging the object.

DAN

That's it. Put it down.

CONNOR puts down the baton. He looks at DAN curiously, then back at his baton.

DAN

Stand still. Hands behind your head.

CONNOR puts his hands behind his head.

DAN

Keep them behind your head. Perfect.

(*to passengers*) All passengers, LEAVE the car. Now. That's it.

(*to CONNOR*) Keep still. Keep cool.

CONNOR

Cool. You, you, you … can see me.

DAN

That's right.

CONNOR

And I can see you. We're the seers. You and me.

DAN

Let them go by. Wait until the car is clear.

CONNOR

The car is clear.

DAN

Okay now – turn around. Walk back toward me.

CONNOR

(*to onlookers on the platform*) They're taking pictures. They're the recorders. The scribes.

DAN

It's just cellphones. It's nothing to worry about.

CONNOR

This … this is a police incident!

DAN

Get off the train. Turn around. Back up toward me. Now.

CONNOR walks very slowly toward DAN, becoming agitated. He goes to pick up his baton.

DAN

Leave it.

CONNOR

I have a job. I need to return to my job. I have information to distribute door to door. People are counting on me.

CONNOR tries to pick up his baton again.

DAN

I said leave it! Back to me. Stop.

DAN walks toward CONNOR.

DAN

Now I'm going to search you. Do you have any sharp things I need to worry about? Any needles?

CONNOR shakes his head. DAN proceeds to pat him down.

DAN

I need to see some identification.

CONNOR

You don't need ID to sit on a fucking beach!

DAN

Watch your mouth. Identification. Now. Slowly. Other hand on your head.

CONNOR produces a letter from his pocket. He very carefully hands it to DAN.

DAN

Hands back on your head. (*reads for a moment*) Connor. Is that your name?

CONNOR

(*recites part of the letter*) "Connor. Your father and I are very proud of the man you have become. We wish you all the best at the University of Calgary."

DAN

Do you have a student card?

CONNOR

Ethan took it.

DAN

Are you here visiting?

CONNOR

WE ARE ALL VISITORS.

DAN

Do you have a driver's licence?

CONNOR extends his hand toward DAN and bows.

CONNOR

VASALON GREETS YOU.

DAN

No comprendes, partner.

CONNOR

(*referring to the letter*) Give that back!

DAN

I'm going to hold on to this –

CONNOR

I need it!

DAN

– unless you can produce some proper ID.

CONNOR

Give me back my letter!

DAN

I told you to keep cool.

CONNOR

That's mine. That's my property!

DAN

Back off.

CONNOR

(*yelling*) I need some help. I need some help now! Push the button! I NEED PROTECTION!

> *CONNOR rushes toward DAN and grabs for his letter. DAN swiftly takes CONNOR down, pinning his hands behind his back and trying to cuff him.*
>
> *CONNOR is terrified. He yells and fights back as hard as he can.*

CONNOR

Help! Somebody ... Get off me!

> *CONNOR manages to get an elbow in DAN's face.*

DAN

Son of a bitch!

> *DAN cuffs CONNOR.*

CONNOR

Get off me! He's hurting me. My head! My head! It's my head!

> *The struggle continues, partially obscured. CONNOR is finally quiet. Blood runs from his mouth and his jaw has been broken.*
>
> *Shift.*

> *Cross-fade to SHARON, that night, on the phone.*

SHARON

He's doing better. He has a job at Student Painters. It's just handing out flyers but I think it's a good sign. Michael and I both said the very same thing. I think Connor likes that it's STUDENT Painters – he doesn't want to lose that connection to university.

I've got a call on the other line. I've got to go, Mum. I'll tell
him. He loves you too. Don't worry. I have to go. He's probably
needing a lift from the SeaBus. I don't want to miss him.

(*switching to the other line*) Hello?

Shift.

That same night. JANIE awakens as DAN enters.

JANIE

You're late.

DAN

I had extra paperwork. I had to talk to Albert. Albert was on
the desk tonight.

JANIE

Tell Albert you'd really appreciate a break on all the nights.
You've got a baby now. How much longer are you on nights?

DAN

I don't know.

JANIE

You don't know your schedule?

DAN

I don't know what day it is.

JANIE

It's Wednesday.

DAN

Fucking nights.

The baby cries out.

DAN

I'll go.

JANIE

Wait.

After a moment, the baby's crying stops.

JANIE

See? He was faking …

DAN

I arrested a kid on the SkyTrain tonight. He had this club
thing –

JANIE

Are you okay?

DAN

He was cracked out or … I don't know what he was. He was out
of his mind. Everybody I deal with is out of their minds. It's all
crazy people fighting with other crazy people. Even the guys
robbing the banks are dinged out.

JANIE

So quit.

DAN

A mall cop does more real police work.

JANIE

Then be a mall cop. You don't have to do this.

DAN

I might as well be a nurse.

JANIE

You could stay home with Zeke. And I could –

DAN

We're NOT getting into that again. I mean it, Janie.

JANIE

I got mad today because –

DAN

And you got mad yesterday and every day last week –

JANIE

– because we can't even talk about it. You won't listen to what I have to say.

DAN

I listen.

JANIE

For four and a half seconds and then you go and hang out with your bike.

DAN

You didn't even like your job when you had it.

JANIE

I didn't like my boss. Or the hours. Or the bus. But the job was okay.

DAN

I'm going to make some toast. You want some toast?

JANIE

I want you to come here.

> *DAN lies down beside JANIE. She wraps her arms around him.*

JANIE

I'm glad you're okay. Are you okay?

DAN

I'm good, Janie. Now I'm good.

JANIE

I've got you.

DAN

I know. I've got you too.

> *Shift.*

Lights up on SHARON.

SHARON

Encounter with the police, number four.

I write down the sergeant's name and Connor's name. Why would I write down Connor's name? And I write down the charges – *causing a public disturbance, resisting arrest.*

I hang up. I phone Connor's dad. Michael's in Seattle on business and will start driving back right away. He tells me to keep calm. And I am calm. I'm remarkably calm.

I get my neighbour, Rachel, to drive me to the station because I don't want to drive. Rachel keeps telling me that everything will be all right. The more she says it, the more I start to feel upset.

How can Rachel know anything? Her twin girls are fast asleep under their twin comforters and all of a sudden I hate Rachel and her adorable little girls.

And then it's like a stink filling up the car. Relief. Rachel is so stunned with relief that her children are just fine, thank you very much, that she ends up getting us lost on the way there and takes us to the wrong station.

Cordova and Gore. Another planet entirely.

We end up circling and circling, checking and rechecking the locks on the car doors, making sure the windows are all the way up. There are a lot of people on the street, hanging out, making deals, shooting up. Dusk, but it feels like the middle of the night there, always.

We find the right station. I wait five hours. No one can locate my son.

Then we find out he's been taken to Vancouver General – the hospital where both his dad and I were born – to have his jaw reset. They bring him back to the station just before midnight.

But Connor doesn't want to see me. Connor doesn't want to see anybody. He just sits there, in hell, in custody for another eighteen hours.

Shift.

Lights up on CONNOR, in a cell, rocking back and forth.

Blackout.

End Act One.

Act Two

Lights up on DAN.

DAN

We've got two high-school kids in the back of the car. They're doing a ride-along for part of the shift – this little Korean girl, MacKenzie, and this big dopey kid with acne, Jackson. They're both in grade eleven. *What made you want to pursue a career in law enforcement?* My partner tells MacKenzie that she signed on because she wanted to make a difference.

Which is what I was going to say.

Before I can come up with something better, Dennis tells MacKenzie that I joined the force because I was good at paintball. I check the rear-view. Jackson comes to for the first time all morning. He writes it down in his notebook – *paintball.*

We get a call about a disturbance at this SRO, this shithole on East Pender. *Single room occupancy, Jackson. You might want to write THAT down.* Before we're even in the building we can hear the wailing. The desk clerk tries a key to a room up on the second floor. We tell the kids to wait by the landing. The clerk opens the door. Furniture upside down, crap – garbage – everywhere. A girl is on the floor, hands tied behind her back, crying away. She's half-naked. I untie her. She's no older than MacKenzie. She's missing a patch of hair on the left side. She's got dried-up blood on her nose and her T-shirt.

She tells us her jeans have been thrown out the window. We send the kids and the clerk down to the alley to look for her jeans. *Who did this to you, miss?* Nothing.

Dennis gives it a go. *It's Sylvie, isn't it?* (*beat*) *We can't help you unless you give us a name, Sylvie. Who do you owe?* The girl stops crying but she's not giving anyone up. Even if she did and we charged the son of a bitch, we'd see him in remand in the morning, then strutting down Hastings by noon. He could have forty or fifty convictions; it wouldn't matter.

The girl – you can smell it on her already. She's gonna end up dead one day, one day too soon.

I don't tell that to Jackson and MacKenzie. I tell them about Janie. How she managed to leave a bad situation. How she took responsibility for her actions and turned her life around. And I tell them about being on the job. How it isn't bad people we're dealing with here, just regular people making bad choices.

Then it's Jackson's turn with the questions. *Have you ever done security on a movie or met anyone famous?* I tell him I pulled over Daniel Sedin once for speeding.

Or maybe it was Henrik. I tell him if I ever pulled over Roberto Luongo I'd lock him up and throw away the key. Jackson writes it down in his notebook.

Shift.

Lights up. Six weeks after the SkyTrain incident.

SHARON enters the police station. DAN rises from his desk to meet her, extending a hand that she refuses.

DAN
Constable Mulano.

SHARON sits down across from him.

SHARON

I know who you are.

DAN

How's it going, Mrs. Crane? Sharon. Can I call you Sharon?

SHARON

I don't care what you call me.

DAN

How's it going, Sharon? What can I do for you today?

SHARON

If you think I'm grateful that after thirty-five phone calls and almost as many requests for information that you've finally agreed to sit down and talk to me, then you're mistaken.

DAN

How's your boy?

SHARON

His name is Connor.

DAN

I remember his name.

SHARON drops a pile of photos and a bound manuscript on the desk.

SHARON

There he is waiting for the school bus, first day of kindergarten. Did he need me to go with him? No, sir. And there's Connor taking home the award for academic excellence in grade eight. All four years of high school he was in the challenge program and on the honour roll. This is the first novel he wrote.

DAN

I was never really much of a reader.

SHARON

We had it bound for his sixteenth birthday. He also wrote a
television script based on the novel.

DAN

Look. I'm not clear what it is you want, Sharon. The charges
were dropped.

SHARON

That doesn't mean someone didn't commit a crime.

DAN

That's correct. Most cases don't get near a courtroom – even
when someone's guilty.

SHARON

And most incidents involving excessive force are never reported.

DAN

I know that you filed a complaint. And I also know that it didn't
go anywhere.

SHARON

The evidence was insufficient.

DAN

The evidence was non-existent.

SHARON

It's all pointless anyway. More police investigating police.

DAN

Look. Mrs. Crane. Sharon. If you had been a passenger on the
train that day and someone was swinging a weapon in your
direction –

SHARON

A weapon.

DAN

– you might see things differently.

SHARON

The so-called weapon was made out of rolled-up flyers from Student Painters that Connor was supposed to be delivering door to door.

DAN

If it's used in a threatening manner it's a weapon.

SHARON

Including objects made of paper?

DAN

If you were a passenger on that train. If you were the one who pushed the emergency button –

SHARON

Connor pushed the emergency button. It was Connor who was feeling unsafe. (*beat*) His injuries have healed.

DAN

I'm glad to hear that.

SHARON

But he's still terrified to leave the house.

> *Beat.*

DAN

I hope he's feeling better soon. I really do. This incident was –

SHARON

This assault.

DAN

Look. He was threatening people.

> *JANIE enters unnoticed.*

SHARON

My son was ill. He needed to be calmed down. He needed reassurance and to have some sense of protection. You treated him as if he were some Saturday-night drunk or petty thief.

43

DAN

You're absolutely right. I didn't give a crap that afternoon that he wrote a book and got a ribbon in grade three. He was a threat to public safety.

SHARON

You're all he's got out there! You and your two and a half hours of training on how to deal with someone in a psychotic state! I want you to think about that the next time you encounter someone in extreme mental distress. I want you to think about Connor.

SHARON turns to exit and comes face to face with JANIE.

JANIE

Dan could've charged him with assault! Assaulting a police officer.

DAN

(*to JANIE*) Go wait out front.

JANIE

You're lucky your kid isn't doing time.

SHARON

Excuse me?

DAN

(*to JANIE*) Not appropriate. This isn't your business.

JANIE

She made it my business. All the shit you said about Dan? The lies in the paper?

DAN

Right now, Janie –

JANIE

Attacking my husband is not going to help your kid. Dan's a good person. And he's perfect – he's a perfect father.

DAN

Go out front and make sure the baby's okay.

JANIE

Denise has got him. Zeke's fine.

SHARON

I hope your little boy never requires surgery. I hope he doesn't
have to get his jaw set and then reset, broken and broken again.
Breaking something again that was already broken seems like
an odd way to go about fixing things, but there you go.

Beat.

JANIE

Dan was doing his job.

SHARON

Connor was on his stomach, on the floor, hands behind his
back. Restrained. And THEN your husband pushed his face
down so hard into the tile that it broke his jaw and four of
his teeth.

SHARON exits.

JANIE examines the photos and the manuscript.

DAN

Just let me sign out and then we're out of here.

JANIE

Are you sure we should go?

DAN

Why wouldn't we go?

JANIE

Zeke's got a cold.

DAN

It's a Vancouver tradition – taking a kid with a cold to the
Christmas train in the pouring rain.

JANIE

    I did Halloween in Stanley Park once – the Ghost Train.

DAN

    Really?

JANIE

    I wasn't in very good shape. (*beat*) Her kid wrote this?

DAN

    I guess so.

JANIE

    I didn't know he needed surgery. Twice.

DAN

    Someone else has this room at four thirty. We've got to get going.

JANIE

    Danny. (*beat*) Tell me –

DAN

    Tell you what?

JANIE

    Tell me whether or not you crossed a line.

DAN

    The interrogation room is just down the hall. You want me to book it?

JANIE

    Those fights about me not wanting to stay home with the baby anymore. We had one of those fights that day. Maybe you carried that into work.

DAN

    I don't carry our shit into the job with me. What do you think we learn in training?

JANIE

You thought he was high.

DAN

He WAS high. He'd smoked some pot.

JANIE

Pot.

DAN

Yeah.

JANIE

Cracked out. That's what you said.

DAN

You're defending him. I can't believe this.

JANIE

Look at the way you treat Bobby.

DAN

My brother weighs three hundred pounds and lives in my parents' basement going through their pension money.

JANIE

He's not having a good life.

DAN

Bozo's not helping my parents have a good life either.

JANIE

You don't even know how to recognize when someone in your own house is depressed. For five months I cried every day and you just wanted to pretend it wasn't happening.

DAN

That's behind us now. You've been doing okay.

JANIE

I still spend half the day just praying that Zeke'll fall asleep.

DAN

That's normal.

JANIE

No it isn't.

DAN

It's just hormones, postpartum stuff.

JANIE

I don't know how to relax with him.

DAN

I'm not listening to this.

JANIE

I don't know how to enjoy him. How can that be normal?

DAN

How can you talk that way about your own son?

JANIE

I don't know. I must be a terrible person.

DAN

So now we sit around and I hold your hand while you tell me about how horrible you are? When's this stuff going to stop, Janie?

JANIE

Never. Once an addict, always an addict. Right?

DAN

What's that supposed to mean?

JANIE

You should've married Denise.

DAN

I didn't want to marry Dennis.

JANIE

Your partner's name is Denise not Dennis. That's not even funny. You should've married someone who's on the job. Don't most cops marry someone who's on the job?

DAN

I married you. I wanted to marry you.

JANIE

And I bet you wish you hadn't. Say it. Say that you wish you married someone different. Say that you wish you married someone different right now.

DAN

I wish I married someone different right now.

JANIE

Fuck you.

JANIE purposely knocks CONNOR's manuscript and photos to the floor.

DAN

That's real mature.

Pause.

Go home, Janie.

JANIE

We're taking Zeke to the Christmas train.

JANIE gathers up CONNOR's things.

DAN

I'M taking him. Get out of here. I mean it. Go home.

Shift.

Lights up on SHARON.

SHARON

One rainy night, at Fifteenth and Granville, after yelling at
customers in a sushi bar, a gifted animator – a bipolar man who
was off his meds – stormed down the sidewalk and through
traffic swinging a bike chain.

Imagine how terrifying it would be if you were in that
restaurant or on that street. At that moment it doesn't matter
that he had been celebrated for his work, loved by his family.
It doesn't matter that for fifteen years he had controlled his
disease. That night his disease controls him – this big, furious
man on a busy street.

Some said that when the VPD showed up, the man ran toward
them. Some said he was trying to run away. He was shot eight
times. I read a theory online that one bullet entered through his
jaw and travelled directly to his heart. The angle the bullet took
when it entered and the trajectory it travelled suggested that the
man wasn't running when that bullet was fired. He was on his
knees – crawling.

My son gets up every day around noon. He drinks the first of
what is probably ten cups of coffee and takes a cocktail of
medication that has changed six times over the past couple of
months – a bit more of this and a little bit less of that – as we
wait it out for some combination of pills to allow Connor to
enter the world again in a more or less rational state.

When he was little, when he was learning to speak – he had this
way of saying the word *squirrel* that made it sound five syllables
long. *Squir-lee-o-o-lol.* I wish I'd made a tape of his voice. Just
that voice. The way his voice used to be.

Shift.

Later that day. CONNOR is writing. He is very hyper.

SHARON enters unnoticed. She watches CONNOR.

SHARON

You're writing. That's great. Is that your novel?

CONNOR types furiously, paying no attention to SHARON.

SHARON

You're going to wear out that keyboard! Connor?

CONNOR continues typing and then finally slams the laptop shut.

SHARON

What was that poem you wrote when Buddy died?

His fur the colour of sun till death was done
His fur the colour of sun till death was done
His fur the colour of sun till *life* was done

I loved that poem.

Pause.

Are you feeling okay? You took your prescriptions and –

CONNOR

Punctuation helps control the speed of speech. It's the poet's friend. Punctuation and Ethan the Mormon. Ethan the Mormon and Punctuation. These are the ones who speak to me.

SHARON checks CONNOR's pill case.

SHARON

You took your pills?

CONNOR

You took your pills?

Beat.

SHARON

I hate that you have to take so many pills. I used to agonize over whether or not to give you Tylenol.

Pause.

CONNOR

Who listens to me?

SHARON

I do.

CONNOR

You don't count. Your opinion doesn't matter in any way. You're not on my radar.

SHARON

Is that so? (*beat*) Were you cuffed when they took you from the station to the hospital?

CONNOR

I don't know.

SHARON

Think about it.

CONNOR

I don't know.

SHARON

Did someone hold your jaw in place on the way there? And were you still bleeding? Profusely?

CONNOR

A red wheelbarrow glazed with rainwater beside the white chickens
A red wheelbarrow glazed with rainwater beside the white chickens
A red wheelbarrow glazed with rainwater beside the white chickens

SHARON

Someone should have been holding your jaw in place in the ambulance. Their inability to do something so basic ... That even the paramedics didn't step in and take charge is simply mind-boggling. Mind you, they're all in cahoots ... I could just kick something.

CONNOR

YOU should be a cop, Mum.

SHARON

I am not an angry person. I have never thought of myself as angry. Even when your dad and I parted company. And believe you me I had plenty I could've been mad about then!

CONNOR

Believe you me.

SHARON

That's right.

CONNOR

You're intense. You're very intense.

SHARON

Let's go for a walk. We don't get out enough.

> *Pause.*

Connor? Do you want a smoothie?

CONNOR

Stop that.

SHARON

I just want you to feel better. You know that. I want that more than anything.

CONNOR

YOU CAN'T COOK! YOU CAN'T DOWNLOAD THE MOVIE! YOU CAN'T BRING THE RIGHT BOOK! YOU CAN'T BRING THE WORDS –

SHARON

It must feel very lonely –

CONNOR

YOU CAN'T TALK TO ME!

CONNOR is on his feet, threatening.

SHARON

Okay.

CONNOR

OKAY? WHAT'S *OKAY*? WHAT DOES THAT MEAN?

SHARON

You're scaring me.

CONNOR backs off.

CONNOR

Do you know what I want you to do?

SHARON

Anything … Tell me.

CONNOR

Stop sucking up all the air in the room. I want you to stop breathing.

Shift.

Later that same evening. DAN is lying down.
JANIE enters.

DAN

You feeling better?

JANIE

Yeah.

DAN

Where'd you go?

JANIE

I came home. And then I was going to go see a movie. I got as far as the bank machine. How was the Christmas train?

DAN

So you hung out at the bank machine for four hours. That sounds like a good time.

JANIE

I hung out at the Starbucks beside the bank machine at the Safeway. I was reading.

DAN

So that's your big night out? Reading?

Pause.

JANIE

The sound that a bank machine makes, that sound it makes when it's getting your money? That is the official sound of getting high. Did you know that? I used to start to feel high when it counted out the cash, just knowing what was coming …

DAN

You should've just stuck your nose up the ATM. It would've saved you a lot of money.

JANIE

It would've saved Jason a lot of money.

DAN

So you wanted to get high tonight?

JANIE

Not a chance.

DAN

That's my girl.

JANIE

I've still got this. Right behind my bank card.

JANIE lays a worn business card on the table.

DAN

That old thing?

JANIE

It's my good-luck charm …

I know you're a good cop. I know you wouldn't hurt someone on purpose. The greater good. You're all about the greater good, right? She freaked me out – the Mother. She freaked me out talking about Zeke and surgery.

DAN

She wants to blame everyone else for what happened to her kid. She should look in the mirror.

JANIE

You think it's your mum and dad's fault that Bobby can't get out of the basement?

DAN

I think my mother babied her baby … She babied Bozo.

JANIE

I feel sorry for the boy. For Connor.

DAN

He's got problems. Mental problems. Don't get me wrong – I wouldn't wish that on anyone. But you know what else he's got? That fuck-you-Jack attitude. He's got that sense of entitlement.

JANIE

He's a teenager. A male teenager. They've all got that –

DAN

It's this city. All the high elevations. All these little shits that grow up on the side of a mountain. Zero respect. They learn from day one to look down on everyone and everything.

JANIE

I read his book.

JANIE pulls out the manuscript and sets it on the table.

The book that Connor's mum left.

DAN picks it up.

DAN

You shouldn't have taken it out of the station.

JANIE

She wanted you to read this book – us to read it. It's sort of hard to follow. But I liked it.

DAN

Volume One. *Vasalon in the Valley of the Clouds*. No, thank you.

JANIE

He was only fifteen when he wrote this one. There're a bunch of them ... It's a real boy book.

DAN reads from the manuscript.

DAN

VASALON LOOKED AT HIS BEAST. SHE HAD ALWAYS UNDERSTOOD HIM IN A WAY HIS OWN SPECIES NEVER HAD.

HER GAZE MET HIS FOR THE LAST TIME AND THEN HER SOUL DEPARTED IN A BLAZE OF GREEN FIRE. HE THREW HER CORPSE INTO A DEEP PIT, WHICH ALSO REMINDED VASALON OF HIS OWN DESPAIR.

You finished this?

JANIE

It's only eighty pages.

DAN

You used to know how to have a good time, Janie.

JANIE

Don't make fun of him. Okay?

DAN ·

Okay.

Lights up on CONNOR lying down. JANIE looks toward him. She reads from the manuscript.

JANIE

VASALON'S HEART WAS HEAVY. HIS BROW, EYES, AND STOMACH WERE HEAVY TOO. HE HAD BEEN TRAPPED IN THE VALLEY OF THE CLOUDS FOR AS LONG AS HE COULD REMEMBER.

YET STILL HE COULD NOT SLEEP.

Shift.

A week later. CONNOR is still lying down, distraught. SHARON enters and sits beside him. Despite her attempts to cheer up her son, she is starting to look more and more worn out.

SHARON

Your dad wants to take you on a road trip. Portland or Long Beach. Or maybe down the Olympic Peninsula. Or New Year's up in the mountains.

I'll bet we did Manning Park ten years in a row. All that snow and then skating outside at night. I loved Manning Park. You did too. You wouldn't have to ski if you didn't want to, but just to get out of here for a little bit. It might surprise you.

CONNOR turns his back on his mother.

SHARON

I wonder if Paul came home for Christmas. You should call his house. Or I could if you aren't feeling up to it. We could invite him over for dinner. I could make ribs. Or risotto. I could make bow-tie pasta. YOU could make bow-tie pasta. Connor?

Five, four, three, two, one – pasta! Again, again! All day. A hundred times a day banging on your highchair, counting down. *Five, four, three, two, one – pasta! ...*

CONNOR cries. SHARON tentatively puts her hand on CONNOR's back. He allows her this.

SHARON

A man who works with your dad has a son – he got sick when he was nineteen. He was at Queen's. And when he was twenty-one he went back to Kingston; he went back to university. This spring he's going to graduate from law school. I want you to hold on to that. I want you to imagine being well again.

I want you to think of your whole life – and this ... right now is just this dark ... this sad chapter in the *Book of Connor*. Right now doesn't define who you are – it's just this tiny little part. By the time you'd turned thirteen, you had outgrown your asthma. This could be just like your asthma. It's unknowable when depression will stop. When you can return to yourself again. A year from now everything could be different. You need to imagine an end, to visualize the end.

CONNOR

That's all I ever do. But I'm not allowed to say it.

Pause.

SHARON

Could you please just try sitting up? Just for a moment? Just for me?

CONNOR

I did it on purpose. I just wanted everything to stop.

SHARON

Did what?

CONNOR

Hurt myself at the SkyTrain station.

SHARON

You were trying to get away –

CONNOR

I wanted to split my head in half.

Beat.

SHARON

You were losing touch with what was going on.

CONNOR

I wanted to split my head wide open. But the cop – he won't let me do it.

SHARON

He smashed your head down on the tile.

CONNOR

He held it tight. He doesn't want my head to break.

Shift.

DAN

The shit list. The ever-expanding shit list.

Crackheads, meth heads, drunks, drunk drivers, junkies, dealers, politicians. Canucks fans. YouTube.

Paperwork. The clerks in Emergency. Welfare day, cold snaps, more paperwork, fireworks. Halloween, New Year's Eve, and every holiday you have ever looked forward to – all on the shit list.

Hookers, activists. Certain strippers. Certain hooker-strippers. Certain hooker-stripper-activists.

Jumpers. Bikers. Street racers. Pig farmers.

Questions you don't want an answer to. *Is this the residence where? Are you the mother of? There's been an incident. There's been an accident …*

Hundreds of things going down that you don't want to hear about and that you don't want to say – day after day after day.

 Shift.

 A week later, JANIE at home. She reads from an invitation. DAN enters.

JANIE
 The circle begins in the east, which represents the child or the beginning. Then to the south, which represents youth. Then the west – adulthood. The circle ends in the north, which represents elders. Participants speak as they pass a talking stick around the circle.

 Did she bring this to the station?

DAN
 It came in the mail.

JANIE
 The invitation looks handmade. I'll bet she did this lettering. Look at the address.

DAN
 What did I tell you? Halfway up the mountain. This is a fucking joke. Honest to god –

JANIE

What if it's a good idea? Meeting with them –

DAN

It's not a good idea.

JANIE

But that's so wild. That they sent an invitation to you – to us.

DAN

They think they're the victims. Jesus, Janie. Don't you get that?

JANIE

I get that. But, I mean, it's called a healing circle. They're inviting us to a healing circle. Not a blaming circle.

DAN

I know all about healing circles. And restorative justice. Do you want to hear my opinion?

JANIE

Not really.

DAN

The Mother probably thinks she's one-twenty-fourth Coast Salish. One-twenty-fourth Native.

JANIE

Her name is Sharon. Not *the Mother*.

DAN

Sharon should hang out with me for a day if she wants to get in touch with that part of herself, with her people.

JANIE

You don't know what her heritage is.

DAN

For a week. Get reacquainted with everybody's despair on a daily basis.

JANIE

Maybe I'll go talk to them.

DAN

Do NOT go and talk to anyone.

JANIE

You don't get to tell me what to do.

DAN

This isn't your problem.

JANIE

Then why did you show it to me?

DAN

I thought it was funny.

JANIE

It's not funny.

DAN

Okay, okay.

JANIE

It's for me too. Family to family. That's what it says. In fancy
letters.

DAN

A real healing circle is through the courts. Just like a real victim
impact statement. She dreamed this circle thing up while doing
yoga and talking to her shrink.

JANIE

We should return his book at least. And the photos and stuff.

DAN

That would be a charming fucking existence, making cards with
fancy letters and dreaming about circles while the rest of the
world is out making a living –

JANIE

I'm going to phone and let them know we can't come.

DAN

Phone. Then we're done with this.

JANIE

Okay.

DAN

I mean it, Janie.

JANIE

Then we're done. (*beat*) How was your day?

DAN

It was nothing. It was a nothing bullshit sort of day. It was one call and then sitting around in the car and sitting around in the station. Which was also exactly like yesterday and the day before that.

JANIE

Your son stood up this afternoon.

DAN

What?

JANIE

Seriously. After his nap. Zeke's standing there holding on to the bars of his crib. Like some demented criminal.

DAN

Get out of the fucking town.

JANIE

Exactly.

DAN

That is so perfect.

JANIE

And you know what? He was proud of himself. I could tell. He thought he was King Shit. And he WAS King Shit. His diaper was bigger than his enormous head.

DAN

Watch out. He'll be running down the hall before we know it.

JANIE

And onto the street.

DAN

Maybe I should just cuff him. Till he's eighteen.

JANIE

Till he's thirty.

DAN

This girl ... This girl OD'd on us this morning.

JANIE

That's awful.

Pause.

What was her name?

DAN

Justine or Céline. Or Cindy ... Something French.

JANIE

Cindy doesn't sound very French to me.

DAN grabs JANIE abruptly.

DAN

Baby numero two. Right now. Put the plan into action. What do you think?

JANIE

I'm not sure the timing is right.

DAN

Go take your temperature.

JANIE

I didn't mean that kind of timing. I'm not ready. Don't push it, Danny, okay?

DAN

Okay.

JANIE

I still can't sleep right.

DAN

I haven't slept right since I joined the force.

JANIE

I'm not saying never ever. I'm just waiting for my energy to come back. It's not personal.

DAN

I SAID I GET IT!

JANIE

Don't yell.

DAN

Okay.

JANIE

You're going to wake up Zeke.

DAN

Okay.

Pause.

Her name was Sylvie. She'd been living down there for the past year and a bit.

JANIE

Sylvie. Do you want to tell me about Sylvie?

DAN

No. I don't want to tell you about Sylvie.

JANIE

Another time. I want you to tell me about her when you're ready. (*listens for a moment*) I think I hear him. Let's go see if he's standing up. (*begins to exit*) Come with me …

DAN

In a minute.

JANIE exits.

Lights up on CONNOR. DAN looks toward him.

Shift.

A week later. CONNOR has his laptop open. He is reading.

CONNOR

THERE WERE NO FENCES AROUND HIS QUADRANT.

THE BORDERS WERE MADE OF LIGHTNING THAT CAME UP FROM THE GROUND AND ROSE TOWARD THE HEAVENS, GREEN AS THE MOSS THAT GREW ON THE GREEN, GREEN TREES.

Lights out on DAN.

CONNOR rises. JANIE enters.

JANIE

Connor?

CONNOR

Yeah.

JANIE

I'm Janie. Thanks for letting me come. You look okay. You're feeling better?

Pause.

JANIE

Look. If you've changed your mind about talking, just give me the word. (*beat*) Here's your book. I like fantasy too. A lot. Like I said on the phone, I just wanted to ask you some stuff about Vasalon's story. His quest. I got really caught up in it.

CONNOR

You can sit down if you want.

JANIE

What a great house. Talk about a quest. I came on the bus, then the train. And the SeaBus. The SeaBus is great. We live in Maple Ridge, out in the valley … Your mum's at work, eh? Did you tell her I was coming over?

CONNOR

It's none of her business.

JANIE

Got it. (*beat*) So … I can't imagine writing an entire book. You made this whole world. A whole universe. Probably most guys your age can't do that. Right?

CONNOR

I don't know.

JANIE

I loved the part when Vasalon was a kid. How he figured out how to do everything all on his own. How to hunt. How to survive. Then, as a man … he's noble.

CONNOR

Yeah.

JANIE

But he's flawed too. I like that. That he isn't just all one thing … Then, near the end, he knows he has to die. He gets ready to die and he sets forth. Right? He sets forth to leave his quadrant.

And for Vasalon, death is okay. He isn't afraid of it. It's this new
beginning and all this new-dawn sort of thing. Right?

CONNOR

Yeah.

JANIE

But it isn't a new beginning. It's the end. Of everything. It's death.

CONNOR

In his world, death is welcomed.

JANIE

It just seems messed up that he didn't have that figured out better.

CONNOR

You're not supposed to like every part.

JANIE

But I didn't think that part was true. And THE TRUTH.
That's a big part of your book. Right?

CONNOR

I guess so.

> *Pause.*

JANIE

So ... my husband, Dan. You probably hate him.

CONNOR

My mum hates him.

JANIE

That's her right. She's okay, your mother.

CONNOR

You don't know her.

JANIE

I know she wanted us to know who you were – so she gave us
your book. And that ... that was a cool thing for her to do.
Then she sent us that invitation for a circle –

CONNOR

I didn't want her to.

JANIE

Maybe she's a warrior, your mum. Like the warrior women that Vasalon befriends in Cloud Valley.

CONNOR

My mother is NOTHING like the warrior women.

JANIE

I guess she wouldn't dress like them. (*beat*) But I mean inside … who she really is … her soul. (*beat*) So here's who Dan is.

She places the worn business card on the table.

When I first moved here, Dan pulled me over as I was coming out of the parking lot at London Drugs. The cops knew the plates. The car was in my boyfriend Jason's name. They were doing some sort of crackdown on stupid guys into stupid shit.

Dan told me my family must feel real worried, me hanging out with a guy like Jason. I was seventeen. My mum and my sister had told me they were worried for me – for my safety – a thousand times. It just never got through.

Dan gives me this card and tells me to give him a call if I ever need help. If I ever want to change my situation.

I didn't do anything for almost a year. But I kept his card. I would take it out and just look at it – four, five, fifteen times a day. And one day I phoned him up. He wasn't partners with Denise yet, but he got me hooked up with this other female cop who found me a place to stay.

And then three years later, I met up with Dan again playing baseball. And the rest, *ta-dah*, is history.

CONNOR

He didn't hurt me on purpose.

JANIE

I know that.

CONNOR

My mum doesn't hate him. She hates the police. She just wants to change the way they do everything. She thinks people like her should be on the police force. It'd be awful.

JANIE

I hear you.

CONNOR

What happened to Jason?

JANIE

He did some time back in Ontario. Then he came back here around the Olympics. Dan's seen him on Commercial, dealing outside the SkyTrain station. But I don't see him. Ever.

So I don't know what your plan is. Maybe it's to go back to school. Maybe it's to go travelling.

CONNOR

Maybe.

JANIE

But if it's ever a plan to die. That's a stupid plan.

CONNOR

I never said that was the plan.

JANIE

Well, your book said it. A lot. And that's in some people. That was in me. And the voice saying that's the plan – it isn't a true voice. Connor. I read your stuff. Your real voice is noble and awesome and cool. Okay?

> *Beat.*

CONNOR

Why would someone marry a cop?

JANIE

  I just told you why.

CONNOR

  You also told me to trust my own voice. Then you won't like
  what I have to say.

JANIE

  Try me.

CONNOR

  Cops are assholes.

JANIE

  Every single one of them?

CONNOR

  Why didn't he come here with you?

JANIE

  Dan's at work.

CONNOR

  Bashing in people's skulls.

JANIE

  Is that supposed to be a joke? Look – I read your book and
  I thought that –

CONNOR

  It's fantasy. Made up. Do you even know what *fantasy* means?

JANIE

  Yeah. I'm not stupid.

   JANIE puts on her coat.

  It must be hard to be so smart –

CONNOR

  Not really.

JANIE

To be so smart and still feel so shitty.

*JANIE exits. CONNOR is still for a moment before
picking up the manuscript that JANIE returned.*

Shift.

*A few hours later. DAN is home, anxiously waiting for
JANIE. She is surprised to find him home.*

DAN

Where's Zeke?

JANIE

You're home early.

DAN

I asked you a question.

JANIE

He's with the Vietnamese lady. I was just going to go get him.

DAN

When did we decide it was okay for him to go there?

JANIE

I decided … I need a break once in a while. I have to look after
myself. If I don't look after myself I can't look after anyone else.
You know that.

DAN

So it's the baby's fault.

JANIE

That isn't fair.

DAN

Where were you?

JANIE

Out.

DAN

Doing what? Come here.

JANIE

I was shoving mountains and mountains of coke up my nose.

DAN

You should've told me about the Vietnamese lady.

JANIE

I tried to, like, eight times. You didn't want to talk about it. (*beat*) I have to be there before five. Come with me. You can see her place. It's really nice. There's lots of toys and stuff. And it's right on the playground –

DAN

Seven months old and he's climbing the monkey bars –

JANIE

I should've talked to you about it. You're right.

I should've talked to you about a bunch of things. (*beat*) I went to see that boy. Connor. That's what I did today.

DAN

Son of a bitch.

JANIE

I wanted to return his book. And I wanted to make sure he was okay.

DAN

So you go spend the afternoon with some fuck-up I arrested instead of looking after your own son? Great plan, Janie.

JANIE

It seemed like the right thing to do.

DAN

Did you make him feel all warm and fuzzy?

JANIE

No. I made a big mess of everything. Like always.

DAN

Here we go –

JANIE

Don't be mad at me. Please don't be mad at me.

> *DAN begins to exit. JANIE stops him and tries to hold him.*
> *DAN remains stiff.*

JANIE

I'm sorry! Danny. Where are you going?

DAN

To get Zeke.

JANIE

I'll come with you.

DAN

No. You messed up. Go have a bath or something. Go make
yourself feel better.

JANIE

I don't know how to feel better!

> *DAN finally holds JANIE.*

JANIE

You've got me.

> *JANIE's attempts to reassure herself don't work.*

JANIE

Are you sure?

DAN

I guess so.

JANIE

I need you to be sure.

DAN

(*without conviction*) And you've got Zeke.

JANIE

I've got Zeke ...

DAN

There's this mum-and-baby-swimming thing at the rec centre. Denise did it when Emma was around Zeke's age. She said it was a blast. You could go on the SkyTrain.

JANIE

I like swimming.

DAN

I need a walk. Zeke and me will go get some sushi for supper tonight. I spent all day inside again.

JANIE

His stroller is at the babysitter's.

DAN

Does that sound good?

JANIE

Yeah ... You'll look after things.

DAN

You got it.

JANIE

You'll always look after things. That's what you do.

DAN

Phone the cell if you need anything else.

JANIE

You're a good man. You're my anchor.

DAN

And that's a good thing. Right?

DAN exits.

JANIE is terrified. She looks toward CONNOR.

Shift.

Half-lights up as CONNOR tears one page after another from his book. He reads from the torn pages.

CONNOR

VASALON PREPARES TO DIE. HE REACHES HIS HAND OUT TOWARD THE WALL OF LIGHT.

JANIE reaches out her hand.

CONNOR

IT'S COOL AS ICE. HE TAKES A STEP FORWARD.

JANIE takes a step forward.

CONNOR

HE FEELS THE COOLNESS ENTER HIS BODY NOW. IT'S AS THOUGH HE IS STEPPING THROUGH A FRAME AND THE UNKNOWN QUADRANT BEFORE HIM IS A PAINTING OF GREAT BEAUTY.

HE SHUTS HIS EYES ...

JANIE shuts her eyes.

CONNOR

... AND FEELS THE COOLNESS TRAVELLING THROUGH HIS VEINS NOW, HIS HEART OPENING ...

SHARON

(*entering*) In Sweden the police are equal parts officers trained in the use of force, social workers, medical personnel, and members from the community. Or maybe it's in Iceland. We should live in Iceland.

Lights up full as SHARON takes in CONNOR sitting amid a pile of ripped pages. He looks up at her.

CONNOR

You should live in Iceland.

SHARON

Is this your book? Connor …

CONNOR

It WAS my book.

SHARON

What did you do? Why destroy something you worked so hard at?

CONNOR

I outgrew it.

SHARON

I didn't. I love that book. Grandma will still have her copy. Are you going to destroy that one too? Should I tell her to put it under lock and key?

CONNOR

I don't care.

SHARON begins to gather the pages. She arranges the torn pages in a pile.

SHARON

I'm going to tape this back together. Some of us are still proud of your accomplishments.

CONNOR

Here's what I accomplished today. I thought about making a sandwich – with your stupid hippie mayonnaise – and how I'll slice the tomatoes thick. But thinking about the sandwich – it's exhausting. So I go back to bed even though I just slept fourteen hours. I wake up two hours later – starving. I eat some Cheerios out of the box. And I watch TV. Now I'm watching you. You and the TV – you're interchangeable.

SHARON

That's a good sign. Waking up hungry …

CONNOR

Stop being a fucking cheerleader.

SHARON

I was too hard on you when you came home from school at Thanksgiving. Your dad was too. We didn't understand –

CONNOR

And stop doing that. Stop going over everything. It doesn't matter what happened or didn't happen.

SHARON

I don't know what happened!

CONNOR sits beside SHARON.

CONNOR

I started getting up earlier and earlier because I couldn't sleep. Because I was afraid I'd be late for class. First class, every class. I time how long it takes to walk between the buildings again and again and again because the time it takes to walk, it changes again and again and again depending on the time of day.

I start thinking the guys who puke in the sinks in the residence on the weekend are doing it to me on purpose. Even Ethan and his nightly calls with his Mormon girlfriend in Cardston, Alberta, are part of the conspiracy.

SHARON

Sweetie –

CONNOR

No. And then one night I'm up on the roof of the residence. It's freezing out. And I have no idea how I got there. I only know there's something wrong with me.

Pause.

SHARON

You're right – this didn't happen to me; it happened to you. That my heart is broken for you doesn't matter. And that you cutting anything with a knife right now fills me with a fear that has no limit doesn't change anything. I will help you make a sandwich. We'll have sandwiches for dinner.

CONNOR

Don't tell dad that I don't know how I got on the roof.

SHARON

Deal. (*beat*) My mayonnaise isn't stupid. It comes from a health food store. It's an organic whole food. Why is that stupid?

Shift.

The next day, JANIE is coming from the ATM at the SkyTrain station, pushing the baby in his stroller. It is the only time we see ZEKE onstage. JANIE is not in very good shape. She talks to ZEKE.

SFX: An announcement. "This is Commercial–Broadway Station. Next train arriving in four minutes."

JANIE

You see, certain people, Zeke, they just can't stand the rules … They can't be held by anything – not even gravity.

So they fall off the face of the earth for a day or a week. Or just for a couple of hours …

JANIE takes the cash out of her pocket and counts it.

Mummy fell off the face of the earth once for an entire year. YOU wouldn't want to do something like that. That would be a stupid thing to do …

Let's go see if Uncle Jason gets off the train.

JANIE releases the brakes on the stroller then freezes. She doesn't know what to do.

> *SFX: An announcement. "This is Commercial–Broadway Station. Next train arriving in one minute."*

JANIE looks back toward the edge of the stage where the tracks are. She slowly turns and walks away from ZEKE toward the tracks. She calls back:

Zeke the freak. Mummy's little man. My boy, Zeke. The biggest boy in the whole wide world.

JANIE continues to walk toward the tracks.

> *SFX: A train approaching. Sound and light grow in intensity.*

JANIE sways forward.

Blackout.

ZEKE wails from his stroller in the black. His cries fade out as the lights come up.

JANIE has stepped back from the tracks. She is sitting on the floor of the station, rocking back and forth, hugging her knees.

SHARON, DAN, ZEKE, and CONNOR have formed a circle – CONNOR at the south point, SHARON at

*the north, DAN at the west, ZEKE, in his stroller, at
the east.*

*They watch JANIE, in the past, still sitting on the floor
of the station, unable to get up.*

JANIE

I'm coming. I'm coming. Mummy's coming …

Shift.

*A month later. SHARON speaks from the circle.
JANIE is still stuck in the past.*

SHARON

When Connor first got sick I told my mother it was as though
an enormous flock of birds had descended on our house.
Blackbirds.

The birds covered the roof – they covered the walls and the
windows. We didn't know where they'd come from – or why.
We didn't know how long they would stay.

Because they'd arrived so quickly, so suddenly, maybe they
would leave just as fast? But that wasn't the way.

DAN speaks from the circle.

DAN

I get the call that she's sitting there, on the floor of the station.
I come right away.

DAN takes a step toward JANIE.

DAN

You've gotta get up, Janie.

JANIE

Zeke –

DAN

He's asleep, he's okay.

I try to help her up. But that pisses her off.

I've got you …

JANIE

No you don't. You are sick of this shit. I am sick of this shit. You are sick of me.

    DAN returns to the circle.

DAN

(*to SHARON*) Janie won't get up.

SHARON

She CAN'T get up.

It happened slowly with Connor. One bird at a time.

He stopped sleeping so much. He was awake a little bit more and he ate a little bit more every day. He started reading again. He hadn't been able to read since Calgary. In March Connor joined an online writing group.

A few weeks later when I came home from work he was at the front door putting on his runners.

    Shift.

    CONNOR sits near JANIE, but they are both in the past, unaware of each other. He laces up his shoes.

    SHARON takes a step toward CONNOR.

CONNOR

I'm going to Paul's.

SHARON

You are?

CONNOR

That's what I just said.

SHARON

He's home for Easter?

CONNOR

He quit.

SHARON

That's good! I mean, not that he quit something, necessarily. But you – go! Have a good time. Say hi to Paul. And to his family. Say hi to everybody from me! Not that they know me that well, necessarily –

CONNOR

Mum. Calm down.

SHARON

Okay. I'm just so happy you're going out. I am happy for you.

> *SHARON watches as DAN goes to JANIE and helps her up. He leads her off, pushing the stroller as they exit.*

> *CONNOR rises. SHARON holds CONNOR tightly then finally lets him go.*

CONNOR

Control yourself.

Shift.

> *CONNOR begins his exit, SHARON watches from the circle.*

SHARON

Connor opens the door. He walks down the front steps. My beautiful eighteen-year-old son steps into the world again. Before Connor disappears down the street, he stops and turns toward me – and I worry for a moment that he's coming back.

CONNOR looks back toward SHARON.

CONNOR
Leave on a light.

CONNOR exits.

SHARON
Always.

Fade out.

End.

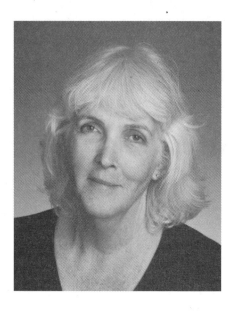

A Betty Mitchell, Chalmers, Dora, Jessie, Governor General's, and Siminovitch Prize–winning playwright, Joan MacLeod grew up in North Vancouver and studied creative writing at the University of Victoria and the University of British Columbia. MacLeod has since published nine acclaimed plays, which have been translated into eight languages and produced throughout the world.

MacLeod developed her finely honed playwriting skills during seven seasons as playwright-in-residence at Tarragon Theatre, Toronto, and turned her hand to opera with her libretto for *The Secret Garden*, which won a Dora Award. She has also had many radio dramas produced by CBC Stereo Theatre, including *Hand of God*, a one-hour drama adapted from her play *Jewel*, and has written numerous scripts for television. She currently teaches at the University of Victoria in the Department of Writing.